Weight Loss tips for a Flat Core:

Core Workouts

Contents

Introduction

Not only does a flat stomach look sexy on someone, it's also a sign that the person is healthy. The fast pace of life in the 21st century and bad diet is the cause of many people struggling with belly fat. In fact, there are more people in the world who are not satisfied with their abs than those who are. If you are looking to make your core muscles look better, then you've picked the right book! Also my website has regular updates on the flat stomach lifestyle at www.losingbellyfatmission.com and free exercise PDF(s) downloads for living healthy.

Losing fat is a long and hard process, but the same was with gaining fat for some. It covers in some cases one's whole life. You may be happy when you were eating sweets and snacks but think of all the harm you are doing your body in the long run. Bad diet and poor lifestyle choices certainly put a lot of pressure on your internal organs such as liver and kidneys, not to mention your heart. Because of all this, losing body fat can create so many benefits for you.

The fact is that it is impossible to lose fat only in one part of the body, so if you go full scale on this, you will improve your overall health for sure. Keep reading the book and find out which are the exercises you should practice daily, which foods are great to help you lose fat, and much more!

Chapter 1 – Weight loss tips

Do not skip breakfast! Appetite can be easily controlled if you have a regular breakfast. Why? The maximum time between two meals is just at night, when we sleep, so between dinner and breakfast may take after 9-12 hours. Now imagine that you skip the breakfast this gap will be spread for a few more hours.

From breakfast, you get calories to work with, even if it was the basal metabolism. Many think that if you skip breakfast that it will make it easier to lose weight, but it is a harmful misconception. In this way, we deprive our body of necessary nutrients early in the day, when the body awakens and becomes active. As a result of skipping breakfast, you will be hungry and eat more food for lunch.

If you think having two meals a day is sufficient for weight loss, you are wrong. By reducing the number of meals you are making a big mistake, because you will eat a lot of food at once. Instead, do the opposite, eat several times, but less, allowing your body to say "everything is fine, do not worry, you'll have enough to eat, you do not need fat reserves." That will accelerate the burning of calories and reduce your craving for snacks during the day. A general recommendation for healthy weight loss is 3 main (basic) meals + 2 snacks in between meals which equals 5.

Eat plenty of vegetables, fruits and grains. Vegetables and fruits are modest source of calories, but an excellent source of vitamins and minerals, but also of, what is very important for weight loss - fiber. Cereals are rich in natural bristles and will give you the energy you need. Fibers accelerate the digestion of food, facilitate bowel movement and remove the feeling of bloating known to many people who want to lose weight. Foods that contain a lot of fiber will keep foods that last a long time, which will reduce the risk of hunger and overeating.

It's definitely confirmed that individuals who introduce physical activity, even if it is minimal, will get thin faster than someone who lives a sedentary lifestyle. Of course, activity has to be adapted to the person holding the diet. The positive experience strengthens the motivation, so it's important that you like that type of workout. In addition to the burning of calories, physical activity has many health benefits.

Keep a bottle of water nearby. Sometimes a person can confuse thirst and hunger, which can negatively affect the weight. If you're thirsty, you do not need juices or sugary/salty snacks, drink a glass of water instead. Daily water needs depend on many factors, but on average, it is sufficient to drink about 2 liters of water a day.

Take a smaller plate. The psychological impact of the size of the plate is huge - if you have a large plate, you'll eat more. Therefore, do the opposite and use small plates, small bowls and small cups. When you see a small amount of food on the plate, you will not be too concerned about it, but you'll get used to it, while still maintaining the same portions. You will not be hungry, but instead will eat it slowly. The brain will receive a signal from the stomach after 20 minutes that it was full, so it's important that you do not eat too quickly.

Do not throw out a whole food group from your diet. Many dieters often throw entire food groups from the diet, which makes us crave them eventually. Moderation is the key, and the amount is determined by the food pyramid. Some pleasures still need to be resolved, but not completely. You can sometimes buy your favorite food, as long as you keep in mind how much you need for daily calories to consume and respect that figure.

Do not buy food with empty calories. To reduce the desire, stop buying snacks, chocolate, cake, crisps and fizzy drinks. Instead, buy healthy snacks, nuts, flaxseed, cereal chips, popcorn and other integral pastime snacks.

Reduce alcohol. Yes, alcohol can make you fat. A glass of wine can have the same amount of calories as a piece of chocolate, a bottle of beer or a one bag of potato chips. As time passes, people who enjoy alcohol gain weight, just from the calories from the alcohol.

Build your own diet. Plan your breakfast, lunch and dinner for at least a week in advance taking into consideration your daily needs and activities, as well as physical and medical characteristics. If this is a bit complicated, is not a sin to ask for help. Take then that menu and go shopping, but do not go shopping hungry, because then you will buy things you do not want. When you are not hungry, it's easier to think. Go online or use a cookbook to get meal ideas if you need to get help planning what to eat. Write down the meals you pick and log at least a week's worth of meal. You can add to your meal list as you come up with and discover new meal ideas.

Remember that diet does not mean starvation, because starvation means overeating and binge eating means obesity. Do not go astray and lose time getting back to the right road. It is not difficult to lose belly fat when you know how.

Chapter 2 – How to Lose Belly Fat?

If you devote each day to regular exercise and proper nutrition, you will never have to stand in front of the mirror and ask yourself, "Do I have to take off some weight?" Once we come to this issue, it's late and the answer is pretty clear. We live in an age where it is not enough to be in good shape, we should be in great shape!

Of course, this is not so easy to achieve - at least not all the time. However, summer is always "around the corner" and we all want to get into shape for summer time. There is no universal solution for removing fat from the abdomen. There are lots of solutions to this problem, but generally if you follow these 10 rules, you'll do well.

1. Eat more protein.

If you thought that this does not have to be pointed out, you're wrong – it's quite the opposite. In addition to being very healthy for your body, proteins maintain muscle mass, while dieting and ensure that you burn nothing but unwanted fat.

2. Compete

You may not have to go out on stage in Speedo trunks and pose in front of 800 people, but you need to make challenges for youself every time you enter the gym. Last time you were doing squats 4 series, now you have complete 5 series. You worked fast walking at an angle of 8 degrees, today increase the angle to 10 degrees and walk for 10 minutes longer.

3. Throw Away Carbs

The best tactic is to eliminate all sources of digestible carbohydrates in the whole two weeks at the start of the diet. This system is so simple, and so it works well when implemented, almost, amazing. Just do not forget your green vegetables - broccoli and lettuce are your best friends.

4. Don't skip meals.

It's amazing how many people today skip meals, all hoping to burn fat faster. This will not only slow down the process of burning fat, but will probably speed up the process of burning your muscles. This is the moment when working out starts to feel extremely hard.

5. Drink more water.

Drink one glass of water before the meal and one glass half an hour after the meal. The glass before meals will reduce your appetite, and the one after will keep you hydrated throughout the day.

06. Avoid snacks

That seductive female voice on TV trying to convince you that their snacks are tasty, and that you'll achieve the ideal shape without dieting, is telling lies! It's better to eat a cardboard box in which the snacks are packaged – it has more valuable nutrients than those snacks. Stick to natural foods you personally make.

7. Do Interval Training

There are plenty of studies that show that interval training is better to remove fat than the classic cardio training.

8. Go by foot.

Whenever you have the opportunity to move some distance on foot use it! In this way, you will increase the overall amount of calories you spend during the day, and I am sure that you will come across some old friends who you haven't seen in a while when walking to places.

9. Chew slower.

People today live faster and therefore eat faster. But that does not mean that food is digested faster. Half-digested food is in the stomach, then gets in the intestines and in the end it just gets thrown away. So, we have less food in the body, the less energy in the system and less protein in the muscles. Just perfect conditions for slowing metabolism and growing fatter.

10. Use a scale instead of the mirror.

Keep the scale in front of the mirror. So every time you step on the scale and see that the pointer is not moved you look in the mirror and check yourself to see if your belly is looking thinner.

Chapter 3 - Best Exercise to Lose Belly Fat

There is an exercise, which melts belly fat, tightens the buttocks, legs, shoulders and arms! It will not be overnight, serious results can be seen after one month, so you need a bit of persistence and perseverance. Here's how you have to practice it.

It is a kind of endurance practice in a position like a push up, which deeply treats and harnesses muscles. This exercise can dissolve fat around the stomach, strengthen the muscles of the torso, but also affect the buttocks, legs, shoulders and arms. All in one exercise!

Begin in a standard position on the floor like you were about to do a push-up. Lie on the forearms, stretch your legs and rely on your toes. The upper body must be a straight line and, while making sure that your hips and buttocks do not drop or, in turn, go too high in the air. Tighten all the muscles and thus control your endurance.

Seemingly it is a simple exercise, but after a few seconds, you will feel that you are mistaken.

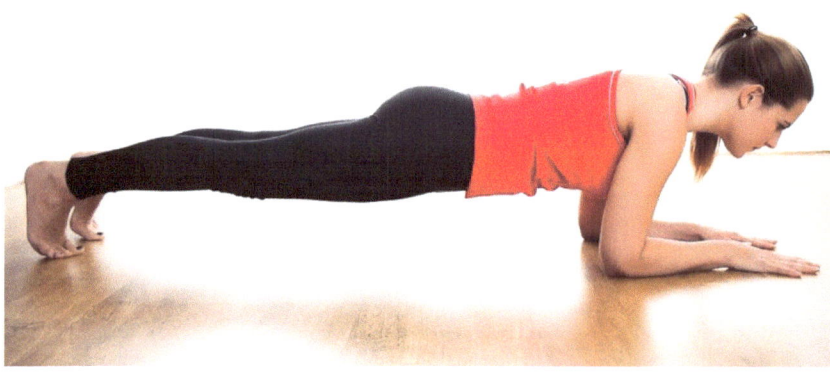

We bring you the schedule challenge boards. Every day, take a little time and a month after admire your new shape!

Day 1 - 20 seconds

Day 2 - 20 seconds

Day 3 - 30 seconds

Day 4 - 30 seconds

Day 5 - 40 seconds

Day 6 - pause

Day 7 - 45 seconds

Day 8 - 45 seconds

Day 9 - 60 seconds

Day 10 - 60 seconds

Day 11 - 60 seconds

Day 12 - 90 seconds

Day 13 - Recess

Day 14 - 90 seconds

Day 15 - 90 seconds

Day 16 - 120 seconds

Day 17 - 120 seconds

Day 18 - 150 seconds

19th day - break

Day 20 - 150 seconds

Day 21 - 150 seconds

Day 22 - 180 seconds

23rd day - 180 seconds

24th day - 210 seconds

25th day - break

26th day - 210 seconds

Day 27 - 240 seconds

Day 28 – as long as you can

Chapter 4 – How to Lose Lower Belly Fat?

Even if you practice a lot the part above the waist is still not what you want. What drives you crazy the most is when the belly fat gets poured over slowly when you sit down. All you want is a super flat stomach on the beach. Well, then read these tips and try to apply them as soon as possible.

You should think about cycling and other aerobic activities. Cycling is one of the best ways to get rid of the fat pads around the waist.

Simply running or riding the bike will not show real quick results, it is better to run at intervals. This training will help in removing fat around the belly (proven). You specify intervals and speed, but be careful not to spare yourself too much from working out hard.

Exercises for more visible muscle tone

In addition to running and cycling, the best recommendation is that you exercise your abs, but also do exercises for the back of the body (the lower back and buttocks). By practicing these exercises you will get leaner and get tighter body shape. Do not skip the workout for the back of your body after you do the abs exercises.

Also, don't avoid going to gym. Push harder and hit bigger weights. The more you lift, the more muscle you will build. The more muscles you have the faster your metabolism will be. Remember muscles burns more calories period, whether at rest or doing an activity.

Remember that neither hard cardio nor spending hours in gym will help you lose belly fat if you don't correct your diet. Diet is the most important thing for weight loss and getting 6 pack abs! Start making changes in your diet after reading the next chapter.

Chapter 5 – Foods That Burn Belly Fat

If you look at food as an enemy that makes you fat, we are bringing you the foods that will inspire you to change your mind. Although any food on the list is good, do not pay attention to only one of them, but to all. Start introducing several new foods that burn fat every week and you'll soon realize that you are eating lot healthier than before.

Tomatoes

Is it fruit or vegetable? Who cares? Everything you need to know is that it contains a lot of good things that will help your body in the long run. The short-term effect will be the weight loss and the prevention of further accumulation of excess weight. Tomatoes contain very few calories, but makes you quickly full and are an excellent source of fiber that help the digestive system. Tomatoes contain lycopene, which has antioxidant activity and for which studies have shown that it helps in the prevention of various conditions and diseases.

Oranges

Oranges are an excellent source of vitamin C, which allows the body to function smoothly. If you want to lose excess weight, you need to pay attention to the intake of oranges because they contain a lot of sugar. Sugar has the potential to be converted into fat by the body. However, the number of calories is really low, and the proportion of fiber to help regulate blood glucose levels is pretty good. To take advantage of oranges, consume them in moderation. Eat orange in the moments when you're craving for something sweet.

Oat flakes

Oatmeal, due to the high share of fibers will accelerate metabolism and will help you feel fuller for longer. Most of the world's experts will agree that a bowl of cereal is the best way to start the day. Oats contain antioxidants and minerals. Reducing cholesterol may also be one of your goals, and oatmeal will help you in this as well.

Spices

No need to eat tasteless food while trying to lose excess weight. This is the right time to start experimenting with spices from other cuisines. Most of them have thermogenic properties that speed up the metabolism, while making the food tasty. Ginger will spice up your meal and speed up metabolism. Use ginseng to increase energy levels, and black pepper to help in calorie consumption. Turmeric may help you in fat breakdown.

Sweet Potatoes

Studies have shown that batat is an excellent substitute for potato, because it contains fewer calories and can make you feel fuller. If you like food that is often undesirable when it comes to weight loss, replace the food such as sweet potato. That way you will enter a lot of fiber, vitamin C, potassium and vitamin B6.

Apples

Apples are so sweet that they can beat the craving for sweets and that is why they are often used in the preparation of desserts. They are an excellent source of fiber. Fiber will keep you fuller and prevent you from being hungry between meals. It will also encourage the work of the digestive system.

Nuts

This is one of the foods contained in the menu of all dietary programs. Only a small amount of raw almonds, walnuts or cashews can be a snack and make you feel good the next few hours. If you are not a fan of nuts, try to chop them and sprinkle the main course with them. This way you will enter the good fats they contain, at the same time enrich the taste of food.

Quinoa

It's great for weight loss and can be used as a substitute for rice, pasta or potatoes. Your dish will still be tasty and filling. You will enter fewer calories and more vitamins. If you still have not tried quinoa, it is definitely time to try it. It will help you feel fuller for longer as it does not contain a lot of calories and has a low glycemic index.

Beans

They are great because they can keep blood sugar levels stable for a long time. Because of the high percentage of fibers, beans will enhance the work of the digestive system. Try to add organic black beans as a side dish to your food and replace bread and rice with them.

Egg whites

The debate over whether eggs are good for losing weight or not, is still on, but most experts point out that the egg whites are acceptable. Eggs are an excellent source of protein. Eat smart and take advantage of eggs by eating only egg whites. When your body weight gets closer to the ideal weight, start bringing the egg yolks slowly back into your diet.

Grapefruit

Grapefruit is probably not on your daily list of foods, but should be. Clinical studies have shown that it can truly enhance weight loss. You can drink grapefruit juice instead of eating it.

Chicken breast

The dark parts of the chicken are not as good when it comes to the quality of protein. Chicken breasts contain little fat and lots of protein. Just remember that you need to eat them skinless. Use a variety of spices to make it tastier.

Bananas

It's very easy to import them into your daily diet because they are easy to take with you. Cut a little banana and add them to oatmeal. They are perfect for those moments when you feel the desire for sweets. Do not eat more than one banana a day because they contain a lot of sugar.

Pears

Pears have a special flavor and hide numerous advantages. They will keep you fuller for a long time, but they have a different consistency of apples and other fruits, which is why their fibers happen to be more efficient. If you don't have a habit of eating pears, now is a good time to start.

Mushrooms

Increase the intake of mushrooms because they contain few calories and are full of vitamins. Experiment with different types of mushrooms, because each of them has its own advantages.

Hot peppers

If you like spicy food, this is definitely good news for you. Hot peppers, such as jalapeno, can enhance weight loss. They contain capsaicin that provides numerous health benefits. If you care about heartburn and think that chili may cause heartburn, you should know that recent research has shown that they can actually help the upset stomach.

Broccoli

Broccoli is truly amazing. In addition to improving your overall health, it can encourage weight loss. Broccoli will fill you up, but will do more than that. It contains a lot of nutritional compounds and is an excellent source of fiber. Season it with spices or hot peppers, but avoid any cheese on it because it will not give you good results.

Green tea

You probably already know that green tea is an excellent source of antioxidants, but did you know that can boost fat burning? This is due to catechins which encourage the body to burn calories faster as well as accumulated fat. Green tea is definitely the best of all types of tea, at least when it comes to weight loss.

Cinnamon

Do not underestimate the power of cinnamon, it is not only to prepare cake and other desserts. Every day, eat a teaspoon of cinnamon and you will quickly notice the results. Cinnamon will help regulate blood sugar levels. It can play a key role in determining how you will feel during the day, how much energy you will have or if you will be tired.

Avocado

Although it contains a lot of fat, these are all good fats. Eating avocado is a great way to assist the loss of excess weight. Avocados will help you spend your stored fat with its high proportion of good fats.

Peanut butter

It tastes great and can satisfy the craving for food. You can add it to a smoothie or smear it on almost any kind of food. Almond butter is also good, but a little less accessible and more expensive.

Salmon

It contains omega-3 fatty acids that promote weight loss and health of the entire organism. Salmon is something you definitely want to eat as often as possible, go for wild caught as opposed to farm raised with any man made additives. If it's too expensive, choose frozen salmon version. Remember that you need very little salmon to make a nutritious and healthy meal.

Olive oil

Olive oil is the best choice of oil for salads with fresh vegetables. Even if you do not change anything else, start every day using olive oil and you will notice first results very quickly. Olive oil is the basis of the Mediterranean diet, which is known to be one of the healthiest form of nutrition in the world. Almost every expert will tell you to start using olive oil.

Linseed

Linseed can be sprinkled over any type of food. They contain omega 3 fatty acids and fiber, which will keep you fuller for a long time. Essential fatty acids speed up metabolism. Another reason why you need to start eating them is that they regulate cholesterol levels.

Eat more soup.

You can make from all your favorite healthy foods a soup. This is a great way to get the most of their advantages, but at the same time enjoy a variety of flavors. Soup is excellent for weight loss. Promotes the work of the digestive system, but it can also work for more healthy foods and thus deliver a perfect meal full of nutrients.

Your favorite soup can be eaten as an appetizer or as a meal late in the evening when your digestive system does not want to overburden. It is easier to digest because of the food in liquid form and in small pieces.

Chapter 6 – Stomach Workouts

Almost everyone have at least small amounts of fat which is positioned on the stomach, regardless of their total body weight. Whether it is a fairly thin person or completely obese one, the stomach represents a place where fat simply loves to get deposited and where it is most difficult to melt.

All this would not have been such a problem if the stomach muscles was not as attractive muscle group, so fat belly can be a real nightmare for a lot of people.

For all these reasons, we bring you a short training program, which consists of three exercises that can be performed at home and that do not require any additional equipment.

You should start practicing these exercises at once:

- Reverse crunches for the lower abdominal muscles (leg lifts, or distorted to avoid injury), 20 reps

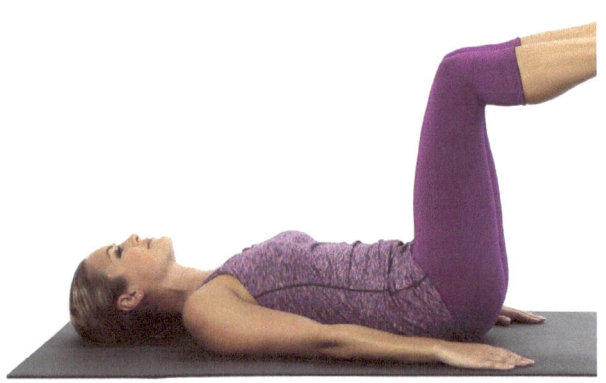

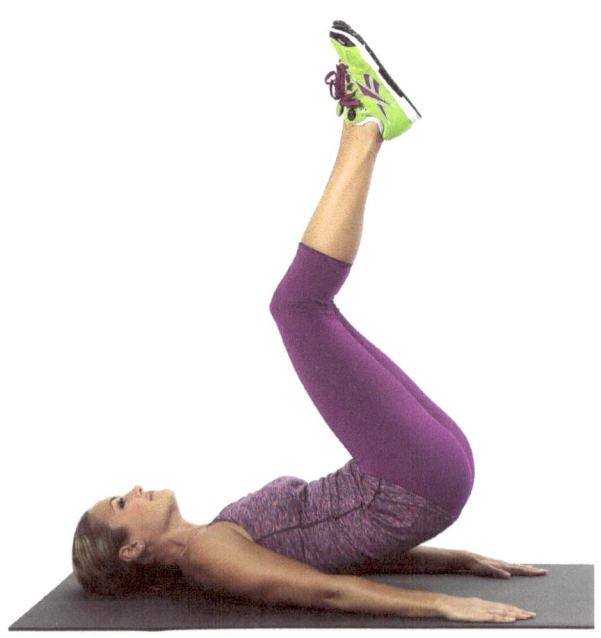

- Abdominal hold will do wonders for your core strength. This exercise will strengthen your arms, lower back, and thighs, not to mention all of your ab muscles. Put your legs up and hold your whole weight with your arms for at least 30 seconds.

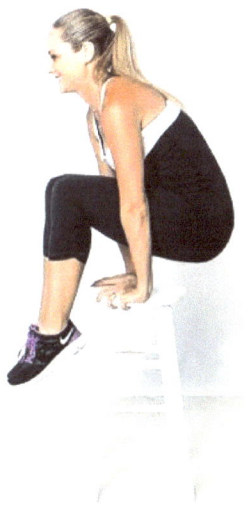

- The hundred is an exercise that is great for every part of the abdomen. It will put pressure on all abs at once. On top of that, it is not hard and most of people can do it easily. Do at least 30 reps per turn.

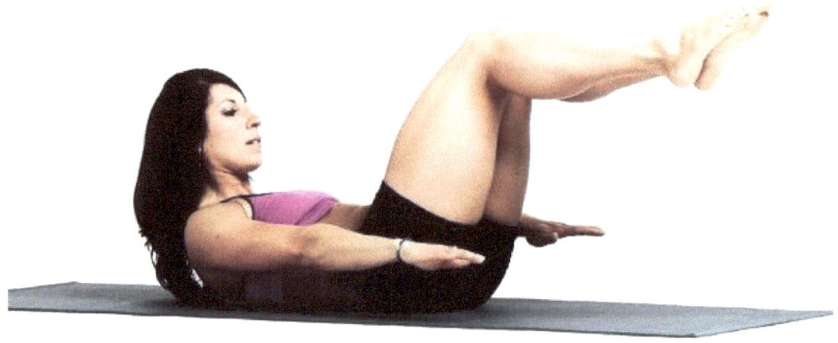

Key to the success of this program is to go through all the exercises without rest, and all of that should be repeated four times!

Chapter 7 – Self Image and Weight Loss

What is beauty exactly is the question that has been on the minds of philosophers and common people alike since the dawn of civilization. The ancient people came up with a formula, the Golden Ratio, but the ideal of beauty is not constant. You definitely cannot calculate beauty as it has trends that are related by many factor. For example, in the past, people with pale skin were considered to be beautiful, while in the 21st century tanned means sexy. A lot of it is popular opinion and culture, it is not exact science and beauty is not constantly one standard either. It is somewhat something more like a moving target. It changes from time to time.

But what beauty is for people is not determined only by time, but also by the place where you live. In some parts of the world, curves are considered to be beautiful, like in South America for example, while Russians and Canada find skinny people more attractive. In fact, the ideal of beauty differs so much and the difference is extreme. Beauty can vary from country to country and person to person within a country. It is largely opinion based, and one's culture can largely influence one's opinion of what is beautiful. Something that is beautiful in one culture or region of the world can be the exact opposite in another region or culture.

Just take a look at music videos of American rap artists and you'll see that they prefer voluptuous women, but if you watch rock videos, you'll see skinny models are more ideal. This shows that some people will find you sexy even if you have a few more kilos.

So, whether you have fat stomach or not is really up to debate. It's all relative, so self image is a way better tool than a scale.

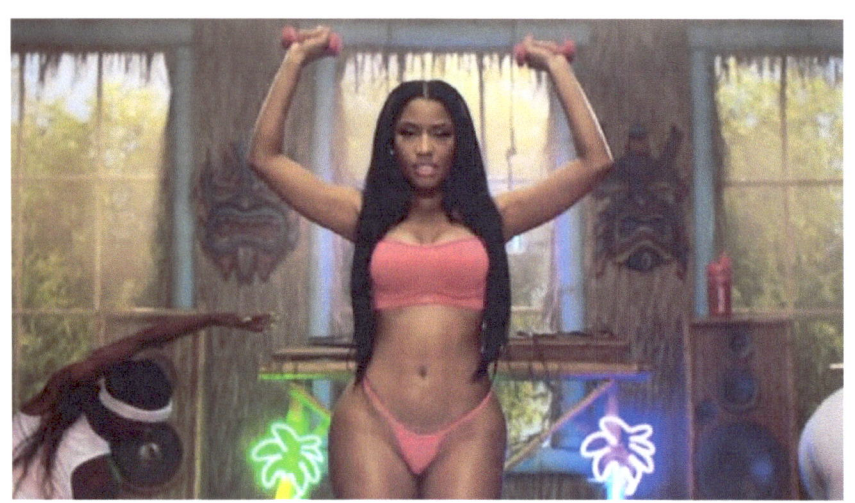

Chapter 8 – Ideal Weight

Determining the ideal weight is not simple mathematics. You need to take so many factors into consideration, from age, height to the level of the activity a person has on a daily basis. The World Health Organization uses BMI, or body mass index for assessing obesity. It is a measurement of body fat using height and weight of the person.

The definition of BMI goes "the body mass divided by the square of the body height". The number you get is your body weight index. The closer to 23, the better. So, let's say you are 1,83m height and have 96kg, your BMI is $96/1.83^2$, which is 28. So, according to the WHO, do you need to lose some weight to get to the BMI of 23, with your ideal weight being 77. In this case, you would need to lose nearly 20 kilograms, which sounds too much.

The reason why BMI is not the best way to calculate the ideal body weight is because of a simple fact – muscles are heavier than fat. That means that an obese person can have the same weight as a slim sportsman. Perhaps it's better to look at the perfect weight the other way, visually.

BODY FAT PERCENTAGE MEN

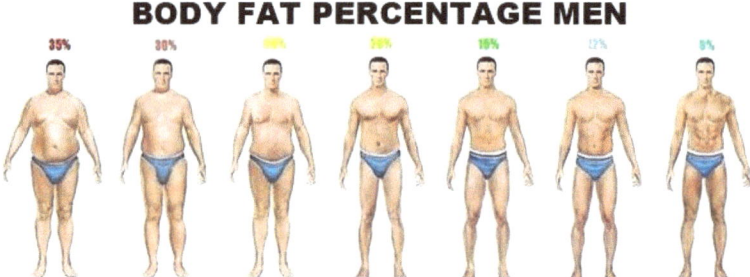

BODY FAT PERCENTAGE WOMEN

| 45% | 40% | 35% | 30% | 25% | 20% | 15% |

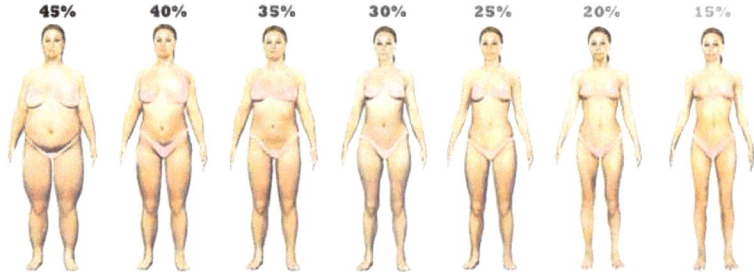

As the image shows, the perfect body is the one with less than 8 percent of body fat.

Chapter 9 – Apple Cider Vinegar Weight Loss

Apple cider vinegar was used in ancient Greece as a medicine while today is increasingly popular as way for losing weight and burning fat. Apple cider vinegar is a natural beverage that is obtained by fermentation of apples that are rich in vitamins and minerals.

Every morning on an empty stomach, drink a glass of water to which you need to add 2-3 tablespoons of apple cider vinegar. The potion is not a pleasant taste and you'll need a little time to adapt.

There are no official data to prove the effect of apple cider diet for weight loss, but there are many positive experiences. There are a lot of factors that influence the positive outcome of the diet, such as for example, body fitness and body mass index.

Many people consuming apple cider vinegar have lost up to 5 pounds in the first month of using it. One should know that the weight loss process is certainly not overnight, but requires sacrifice and of course exercise.

Conclusion

Don't expect that if you follow the advice from this book, you will lose fat in only a few days. Burning belly fat is a process that takes a while. In fact, it should never end. The stomach is an area that easily gets fat accumulation. To make things even worse, the belly is one of the most noticeable parts of the body.

Because of this, you need to work hard and make working out a part of your everyday life to win both the battle and the war of the midsection bulge. But, that will not matter much if you get back to eating snacks and sweets. The only way you'll manage to stay fit and look awesome is by changing the lifestyle, from lazy to active.

That is why this book should be your guideline for the future. Do not forget about it once you get into the desired shape as you will probably need it again at some point in the future. Again, you can visit my website for regular diet and exercise tips there at www.losingbellyfatmission.com and see your dream body come to fruition. If you like this type of topic this is the website to go to for regular exercise blogs, and subscribe there to get access to a lot of good exercises workout tips. Also feel free to check out some of my other ebooks at Amazon and Createspace, under my primary author name: Oswin Dacosta, anytime. Thanks for picking up my book.

www.ingramcontent.com/pod-product-compliance
Lightning Source LLC
Chambersburg PA
CBHW050929290526
45792CB00002B/938